THE COMPLETE GU USE PRILIGY

The Beginners Guide to Effectively Treat Premature Ejaculation(PE), Increase Ejaculation Timing,Reduce Distress and Anxiety Over Ejaculation and Make Her Never Leave You

ISBN 978-1-387-38531-7

Harrison Daly

TABLE OF CONTENT

CHAPTER 1
BASICS OF PRILIGY

PRILIGY is a drug that might be beneficial to you if you are a guy between the ages of 18 and 64 and suffer from any of the following symptoms of premature ejaculation (PE).

ejaculating less than two minutes after vaginal penetration, often without any encouragement and in advance of the guy's desire; and ejaculating when the man is still wanting more.

An untimely ejaculation may create severe mental distress as well as difficulties in interpersonal communication for both the man and his partner.

PRILIGY is a drug that is categorized as a selective serotonin reuptake inhibitor (SSRI) and is used as a therapy for urological conditions. The active component of PRILIGY is dapoxetine. The amount of time it takes to ejaculate is increased with PRILIGY, which may lead to more control and a reduction in concern around ejaculatory frequency and volume. It's probable that this may make you feel more satisfied after sexual interactions thanks to this.

Make it a point to inquire about the reasoning behind your prescribed medicine with your primary healthcare provider if you're interested in learning more.

There is a possibility that your physician prescribed it for some other purpose.

In order to purchase this drug, a doctor's prescription is required.

Be very careful while taking PRILIGY!

CHAPTER 2
WHEN NOT TO USE PRILIGY

When it is really essential to miss up on the opportunity

You should not use PRILIGY if you have ever had an allergic reaction to dapoxetine or any of the other ingredients that make up this drug.

Rash, itching, and hives on the skin are some of the external manifestations of an internal allergic response. Difficulty breathing, wheezing, or shortness of breath may also be symptoms of an allergic reaction. Swelling of the face, lips, tongue, or other areas of the body is another possible symptom of an allergic reaction.

Do not use PRILIGY if you are now on or have recently ceased taking a monoamine oxidase inhibitor (MAOI), such as those used to treat depression. This includes patients who have recently completed treatment with an MAOI (see Taking other medicines for examples of MAOIs). After you have stopped taking PRILIGY, wait 7 days before beginning treatment with an MAOI.

Wait 14 days before moving further if you are currently using the anti-schizophrenia medicine thioridazine or if you have just stopped taking it. Before beginning treatment with thioridazine, you should wait seven days after finishing your last PRILIGY dosage.

If you are currently taking a serotonin reuptake inhibitor or have taken one within the past 14 days, you should not take this medication. Examples of serotonin reuptake inhibitors include selective serotonin reuptake inhibitors (SSRI), serotonin-norepinephrine reuptake inhibitors (SNRI), tricyclic antidepressants (TCA), and certain other medications and herbal products to treat depression (see Taking other medicines for examples of serotonin reuptake inhibitors and other medicines used to treat depression). After you have stopped using PRILIGY, you should wait a full week before beginning treatment with any of the medications or supplements listed above.

You could have this side effect if you are using medication for the treatment of HIV/AIDS or a therapy for fungal infections (see Taking other medicines for examples of these medicines).

In the event that there is a history of either manic or depressive episodes in the patient's past

PRILIGY is not something you should take if you have any kind of cardiac condition, such as heart failure or an abnormal heart rhythm.

You should not take PRILIGY if you have any degree of liver disease, whether it be mild, moderate, or severe.

You should not take PRILIGY if you have a history of fainting or dizziness due to low blood pressure because of the risk that it poses (Syncope).

Patients under the age of 18 or above the age of 65 are not eligible to utilize PRILIGY.

Patients under the age of 18 and patients over the age of 65 have not been thoroughly investigated to establish whether or not the treatment is safe and effective for these age groups.

It is strongly recommended that females do not participate in PRILIGY.

Investigations have been conducted to determine whether or not PRILIGY is beneficial in treating premature ejaculation in men. We are unable to determine whether or not it is risky for women to use.

It is imperative that attention be given to the fact that this prescription contains lactose (a type of sugar). If your physician has advised you not to consume particular sweets because you have a sugar intolerance, you should not use this prescription.

You should avoid taking this medicine if the date on the box indicates that it has expired or if the box seems to have been tampered with.

If it's damaged or beyond its expiration date, bring it back to the pharmacy so they can dispose of it.

If you are unsure about starting this therapy, you should discuss your concerns with your primary care physician.

Hold off till you've already begun taking it.

Before giving you this medicine, your physician should check your blood pressure after you get out of a sitting or lying position and immediately after you stand back up.

If you experience any of the following symptoms and have not been diagnosed with premature ejaculation, it is imperative that you see your primary care physician immediately: If you are allergic to any other drugs, foods, preservatives, or colors, then you should not use this medication.

You are a user of ecstasy or LSD who enjoys going out to parties (lysergic acid diethylamide). Patients who used PRILIGY in conjunction with these other drugs had a heightened risk of serious adverse reactions.

You may choose to medicate with opioids, which are very potent medications, or benzodiazepines, such as Valium. The sedative and vertigo-inducing effects of PRILIGY may be heightened when used with these other medications.

You're drinking. Consuming alcohol while taking PRILIGY significantly increases the risk of losing consciousness.

Your depression is being treated, which is wonderful news.

You are currently taking medication that combats fungal infections.

You are using blood-thinning medicine such as aspirin, anticoagulants such as warfarin, non-steroidal anti-inflammatory medications (NSAIDs) such as ibuprofen, or mental drugs such as antidepressants, all of which have the potential to induce bleeding. It is possible that serious bleeding issues will emerge when PRILIGY is combined with the usage of certain other medications.

Please contact your doctor if you are presently experiencing any of the following medical concerns or if you have ever had any of these problems in the past:

Background of lightheadedness caused by low blood pressure, difficulties with the heart and blood vessels, anemic condition, history of fainting, or depression (see Things to be wary of) you're considering harming yourself or taking your own life.

If you are experiencing thoughts of suicide or any other form of mental or emotional upheavals, you should contact your primary care physician or a mental health professional as soon as possible.

a history of manic episodes (great excitement, hallucinations, difficulty concentrating or remaining still) or bipolar illness (extreme mood fluctuations between mania and depression); the start of these conditions. seizures (fits) or have uncontrolled epilepsy.

abnormalities of the liver, renal illness ranging from moderate to severe to critical, and other sexual issues such as erection dysfunction. It is uncertain at this time whether or not PRILIGY may make these symptoms worse.

a condition affecting the eyes, such as glaucoma (also known as excessive pressure in the eye), or HIV;

If you have any of the illnesses or symptoms listed above and have not previously done so, you should make an appointment with your primary care physician before commencing treatment with PRILIGY.

CHAPTER 3

EFFECTS OF OTHER DRUGS ON PRILIGY

Inform either your primary care physician or your pharmacist if you are currently taking any extra prescriptions, including any that you have obtained from an over-the-counter section of a pharmacy, grocery shop, or health food store.

It's possible that PRILIGY might have a harmful interaction with other drugs. Some examples of MAOIs that are used in the treatment of depression are moclobemide, phenelzine, and tranylcypromine.

antidepressants include amitriptyline, citalopram, escitalopram, doxepin, fluoxetine, fluvoxamine, mianserin, mirtazapine, nortriptyline, paroxetine, sertraline, nefazodone, venlafaxine, and vortioxetine.

medications for migraines, such as sumatriptan and rizatriptan; painkillers, such as tramadol; lithium, a prescription used to treat mental illness

The use of thioridazine in the treatment of schizophrenia.

antimicrobial medication used in the treatment of infections that is analogous to linezolid.

It's possible that the amino acid tryptophan may lift your mood and make it simpler for you to go to sleep.

St. John's wort is a natural treatment for mental health conditions such as depression and anxiety (Hypericum perforatum)

If you are currently using any of the medications or herbal supplements on this list, or if it has been less than 14 days since you stopped taking any of those medications or supplements, you should not take PRILIGY.

After you have stopped using PRILIGY, you should wait 7 days before beginning treatment with any new drugs or herbal supplements.

It is possible that the effects of PRILIGY will be diminished if it is used in conjunction with certain meals or drugs. Medication for disorders other than depression is one example of this.

Warfarin, ketoconazole, itraconazole, and fluconazole are some examples of anti-fungal medications. Other examples include pharmaceuticals that are used to thin the blood, such as fluconazole.

Anti-inflammatory drugs like ibuprofen or aspirin, which may cause a drop in blood pressure, potentially upon standing Certain anti-HIV medications, such as ritonavir, saquinavir, and atazanavir Certain pharmaceuticals used to treat high blood pressure and chest discomfort (angina), an enlarged prostate, or erectile dysfunction (impotence), due to the fact that these medicines may lower your blood pressure Certain pharmaceuticals used to treat high blood pressure and

Antibiotics, such as erythromycin, telithromycin, and clarithromycin, are often used in the treatment of infections.

Aprepitant is effective in alleviating nausea.

grapefruit. Grapefruit juice should not be consumed for at least 24 hours before or after using opioids (medications used to treat severe pain) or benzodiazepines like valium. The sedative and vertigo-inducing effects of PRILIGY may be heightened when used with these other medications.

alcohol. Consuming alcohol while taking PRILIGY significantly increases the risk of losing consciousness.

Visit your primary care physician or local pharmacy if you are unclear whether or not you are already taking any of these drugs.

The presence of these other medications may have an impact on the therapeutic efficacy or adverse effects of PRILIGY. It's possible that changing the dose or trying a different medicine may be required.

It is possible that PRILIGY may interact with other drugs or reduce the efficacy of other treatments. Consult your primary care physician or local pharmacy for further information on the medications that you should steer clear of or take with extreme caution.

CHAPTER 4
TAKING PRILIGY INFORMATION

Always be sure you thoroughly read and adhere to the directions provided by your pharmacist or doctor.

It's possible that they're not the same as what's described here.

Is there anybody who can tell me how much of this substance I should take?

It is recommended to take one tablet (30 mg), as required, between one and three hours before engaging in sexual activity.

Take only one tablet per day at most.

Knowing when to take it easy and when to power through it is essential.

When taking the tablets, it is recommended that you drink at least one full glass of water to mitigate any potential harshness.

Taking PRILIGY with or without food does not affect how well it is tolerated by the body.

Do not consume any alcoholic beverages while taking PRILIGY.

If you have had grapefruit juice within the last 24 hours, you should not take PRILIGY.

If you take this medication together with grapefruit juice, there is a possibility that the drug's concentration in your system may increase.

When to Take Your Dose

When required, take the pill between 1 and 3 hours before participating in sexual activity. Generally, this should be done between 1 and 3 hours before.

In the event that sexual activity is intended to take place, PRILIGY may be necessary. When used on a regular basis, you should not expect it to endure.

It is best not to take more than one tablet in a 24-hour period since doing so puts you at greater risk of negative effects and provides no additional benefit.

Even if you skip a dosage

Given that PRILIGY is an as-needed drug, skipping a dosage of it will not result in any adverse effects.

The possibility of receiving an excessive dosage rises (overdose)

If you believe that you or someone you know may have taken an excessive amount of PRILIGY, get immediate medical attention by contacting either your primary care physician or the Poisons Information Centre at 13 11 26 (Australia) for direction. Do not wait until you are in pain or start experiencing signs of poisoning before doing this.

Notify your healthcare provider or pharmacist as soon as possible if you discover that you have taken a higher dose of PRILIGY than what is suggested for you. It's likely that you may become ill or sick. Overdosing on PRILIGY may cause a variety of unpleasant side effects, including weakness, nausea, vomiting, agitation, tremors, and disorientation. If you believe that someone has taken too much PRILIGY, you should seek emergency medical attention right away. This is a severe situation.

A word of caution: taking PRILIGY can make you feel dizzy or cause you to pass out while you're doing it.

In order to reduce the possibility of anything like this occurring, the following precautions should be taken:

It is recommended that PRILIGY be consumed together with a full glass of water.

You should not take PRILIGY if you are dehydrated at the time of your dose (you do not have enough water in your body).

You have gone four to six hours without drinking anything, which may have occurred if any of the following was true:

Your sweat has been rising steadily for a considerable amount of time now.

You've been struck down by an illness, and as a result, you're either running a fever or vomiting up, or both.

You're definitely inebriated.

If you feel faint, lightheaded, or dizzy, or if you feel weak, confused, sweating, or have an irregular heartbeat, or if you feel dizzy when you stand up, lie down so that your head is lower than the rest of your body, or sit with your head between your knees, and remain in that position until you feel better.

If you feel weak, confused, sweating, or have an irregular heartbeat, or if you feel dizzy when you stand up, lay down so that your head This will prevent you from falling and injuring yourself if you are feeling dizzy or faint.

Take your time while rising up after being seated for a long time or lying down for a prolonged length of time.

If you experience dizzy while taking this drug, you should avoid driving, using tools, or operating equipment.

Tell your doctor right away if you start to feel lightheaded or faint while you are on this medicine.

Essentials to remember

Before beginning treatment with any new medication, you should inform both your primary care physician and your pharmacist that you are currently taking PRILIGY.

It is important that you discuss the fact that you are taking this medicine with both your primary care physician and your dentist.

Make it a point to attend each and every one of your doctor's appointments.

Do not stop taking this medicine suddenly without first discussing it with your primary care physician. Even if you haven't been taking it on a regular basis, you may still have withdrawal symptoms after you stop using it, such as sleeplessness and dizziness.

Steer clear of engaging in these activities!

You shouldn't use PRILIGY if your physician hasn't recommended it to treat a particular condition related to your health.

Under no circumstances should you ever give another individual your medicine, not even if they suffer from the same condition as you do.

CHAPTER 5

Precautions That Should Be Taken

Take precautions before using potentially dangerous machinery or driving until you have a better idea of how PRILIGY will impact you.

This medicine may cause a number of unpleasant side effects, including but not limited to feeling faint or dizzy, exhaustion, drowsiness, difficulty concentrating, and impaired vision. If you are feeling any of these symptoms, it is imperative that you refrain from operating any machinery, driving a vehicle, or participating in any activity that might put you or others in danger.

Do not consume any alcohol while you are under the influence of this medicine.

When used with PRILIGY, the negative effects of alcohol consumption—including drowsiness, slowed reflexes, and impaired judgment—may become even more pronounced.

Check to see whether your body is suffering from a lack of adequate water levels (dehydrated).

If it's been more than four to six hours since you last drank anything, if you've been heavily sweating, or if you have a disease that causes you to sweat excessively, have a high body temperature, or throw up, this could happen to you. Other factors that could cause this include heavy sweating, a high body temperature, and excessive sweating.

When taking PRILIGY, it's conceivable that you might pass out. It is recommended that PRILIGY be taken with at least one full glass of water in order to lessen the likelihood of passing out and the damage that may accompany it.

Instead of putting yourself in danger by falling because you are dizzy or fainting, you should lie down as soon as you feel any of these symptoms.

After using PRILIGY, you should avoid getting up too quickly from a sitting or reclined posture too soon after taking the medication.

If you are having any of these symptoms, it is not safe for you to operate heavy equipment or drive a vehicle.

Results That Have Their Downsides

If you start to feel unwell while you are taking PRILIGY, you should contact your healthcare provider or pharmacist as soon as possible.

Even though this drug is typically well-tolerated, there is always a possibility that some individuals may have unfavorable side effects. Every drug has the potential for causing side effects. They sometimes show signs of being serious, but for the most part, they are not. If you have particular unfavorable consequences, you should probably see a physician.

The following list of potential adverse effects includes some that are less severe than others. There is always the chance that none of these things will take place to you.

If you have any questions or concerns, you should consult with either your physician or your pharmacist as soon as possible.

While using PRILIGY, you should get in touch with your physician as soon as possible if you experience any of the following unwanted effects: if you have fits (seizures)

Make an appointment with your primary care physician or pharmacist if you are concerned about any of the following issues.

nausea

headache \sdizziness

Do not put off going to the doctor if you encounter any of the following symptoms; do so as soon as possible:

experiencing lightheadedness or fainting upon standing (see While you are taking PRILIGY)

Symptoms of shaking, tingling, or numbness might be caused by an increase in blood pressure.

hazy perceptions

earaches and eye strain are also present.

Clogged nose

Erectile dysfunction, fatigue, tiredness, irritability, difficulties paying attention, and yawning are only some of the symptoms. Other symptoms include diarrhea, stomach pain, dry mouth, vomiting, indigestion, intestinal gas, constipation, bloating, and excessive sweating (difficulty getting or keeping an erection)

Mental health conditions such as anxiety, irritability, poor libido, depression, and apathy are examples of these

irregular dreaming

irregular bleeding and bruising

Immediately contact your primary care physician or the emergency department of the nearest hospital if you have any of the following symptoms:

Common allergy symptoms include swelling of the face, lips, tongue, or other areas of the body; difficulty breathing; a rash, itching, or hives on the skin; and other skin reactions.

If you are ever feeling unwell, it is imperative that you contact either your doctor or your pharmacist.

It's possible that some people will have repercussions in addition to those stated above.

After PRILIGY Storage has been put to use

Do not bother removing the pills from the bag until it is the appropriate moment to do so.

If you take the tablets out of their package, they may not keep as well.

Tablets should be kept in a dry environment that does not exceed 25 degrees Celsius and should be kept at a cool temperature.

It is important to keep PRILIGY out of the bathroom and away from the sink so that it does not get contaminated. You shouldn't simply leave it on the seat of the car or on the window ledge.

If a certain medication is damaged by either heat or moisture, it cannot be fixed.

Put it in a location where children can't get to it.

At a minimum of 1.5 meters above the ground, medicines should be stored in a cabinet that can be locked.

Disposal

If your physician has directed you to discontinue taking a certain drug, you should probably talk to your pharmacist about what you should do with any leftover medication.

Explanation of the Content of Question

How it seems to be.

PRILIGY 30 mg film-coated tablets are available. These tablets are light gray in color, circular in shape, and marked with the number "30" inside of a triangle.

Tablets of PRILIGY may be purchased in blister packs containing either three or six tablets.

Ingredients

The active ingredient in PRILIGY is dapoxetine hydrochloride, and each dosage of the medication is 30 milligrams.

In addition, there is lactose monohydrate included in the components.

microcrystalline cellulose

croscarmellose A particle suspension consisting of an anhydrous sodium silicate, stearic acid, magnesium hypromellose, and iron oxide. titanium dioxide Yellow oxide of iron (which is black) striacetin

This drug does not have any added sugar or gluten, and it does not contain any azo dyes either.

CHAPTER 6

PRILIGY EXPLAINED IN FEW LINES

There is a lot of confusion around Priligy; could you kindly elaborate?

A drug called Priligy is available for use in the treatment of premature ejaculation. Dapoxetine, which is the principal component of this medicine, is a member of a class of pharmaceuticals known as selective serotonin reuptake inhibitors (SSRIs). Men between the ages of 18 and 64 who are suffering premature ejaculation are the target demographic for this medication. Men who ejaculate before the appropriate time may be able to make their sperm remain in their system for a longer amount of time with the assistance of Priligy.

The very best of the best

What specific advantages does Priligy have to offer?

The active component of Priligy, dapoxetine, achieves its effects by inhibiting the reuptake of serotonin (short-acting selective serotonin re-uptake inhibitor). The hormone serotonin is responsible for controlling a wide variety of biological activities, one of which is the rate at which you ejaculate. As a result of Priligy's ability to raise serotonin levels in the neurological system, the pace at which the brain receives impulses to ejaculate is slowed down. This will increase your endurance and allow you to play for a longer period of time.

When I take Priligy, what kinds of results should I expect experiencing?

Because of the quick onset of action after consumption of Priligy, it is recommended that you take the medication anywhere from one to three hours before you intend to engage in sexual activity. It is typical for the onset of symptoms to be delayed or advanced for some people, so there is no need for you to worry about this. This varies from person to person.

Is there any truth to the Priligy hype?

Men who use Priligy for the treatment of premature ejaculation report positive results in eight out of ten cases. In the clinical trials of Priligy for males with premature ejaculation, positive results have been observed, with some men claiming that their erection length increased by a factor of three.

The very best of the best

Always be sure to take Priligy exactly as directed.

It's possible that the regular 30-milligram pill of Priligy isn't the safest amount for you to take, and that your doctor will recommend instead that you take 60 milligrams instead. Consume the pill anywhere from one to three hours before you want to have sexual activity. It is strongly advised that Priligy not be used more than once a day at a time. When you take the pill, be sure to drink a full glass of water at the same time. It is up to you whether you take it before or after eating.

When Should Priligy Be Taken?

Taking Priligy anywhere from one to three hours before engaging in sexual activity is recommended. Take care, and make sure you don't go over the daily limit that's suggested.

How much of the medication must be taken before it begins to have an effect?

The typical dosage is 30 milligrams, although in more serious circumstances, 60 milligrams may be required. Talk to your healthcare provider if you feel as if you need a greater dosage than what was recommended for you.

When should Priligy be taken and how long should each dose be?

Long-term treatment with Priligy may be able to prevent premature ejaculation, but you will need to see your doctor somewhat often. After taking Priligy for a total of 6 times or after 4 weeks of treatment, a trip to the doctor is advised. By carrying out these steps, they will be able to determine if the current dosage is enough or whether adjustments are required. As part of the

Superdrug Online Doctor service, our experts will consult with you and ask you some fundamental questions on your therapy as well as any potential adverse effects you may be experiencing.

The very best of the best

Where would it be feasible for me to get Priligy?

If I decide that I want to purchase Priligy, is it possible for me to do so online?

There are reputable retailers, such as Superdrug Online Doctor, where you may purchase Priligy. Just a few minutes of your time to fill out a brief and confidential online form is all that is required from you in order for one of our medical professionals to evaluate your case.

If it is determined by your doctor that you might benefit from this treatment, we will happily fill the prescription that he or she writes for you, and you will then be able to buy the therapy from our online store. There will be no out-of-pocket costs associated with the delivery of Priligy to your house, and the procedure of delivery will be carried out in a manner that is totally confidential. You won't need a prescription to get Priligy, and you can pick it up at any local Superdrug.

Have you heard whether or not Priligy may be purchased without a prescription from a medical professional?

Because Priligy may only be obtained via a doctor's office or the pharmacy of a hospital, you will be need to have a prescription in order to purchase it. If you don't already have a prescription, you may either go to your family physician or make advantage of the easy-to-use online doctor service that Superdrug provides.

I'm wondering whether the National Health Service will pay for my Priligy prescription.

However, Priligy is not covered by the National Health Service (NHS) in all regions. This indicates that your physician probably won't suggest it unless there are very specific conditions present.

The very best of the best

What You Need to Know About Priligy and Why It Isn't the Right Choice for Everyone

Some people who use Priligy could have unfavorable side effects from the medication, however this is not always the case. While using Priligy, if you experience any of the following, you should contact your healthcare provider as soon as possible: experiencing lightheadedness or vertigo when standing Stop using it right now and get medical help as soon as possible.

If you suffer any of the following unwanted side effects while using Priligy, you should immediately seek medical attention and stop taking the medication.

If you are experiencing suicidal thoughts or emotions, or if you witness any unusual bleeding (including bloody vomit), facial swelling, or trouble breathing, make a huge deal out of nothing (a seizure).

The following are some instances of typical unfavorable reactions:

headache

having problems with both dizziness and nausea

Nausea and a blurring of vision are common adverse effects that might occur.

a reduction in sexual desire when in bed.

persistent ear noises

alterations in one's emotional state, such as a heightened sense of irritability or anxiousness, numbness, or tingling.

Symptoms such as trembling, hypertension, nasal blockage, fatigue, yawning, sleeplessness, and odd dreams are all associated with this condition.

Discomfort and fullness in the stomach that makes one queasy and want to vomit up (being sick)

Problems with irritable bowel syndrome (also known as IBS), diarrhea, and constipation heat and wind might make it difficult to get or maintain an erection.

oral and lingual tissues become more dehydrated

Fainting, dizziness on standing, feelings of extreme excitement or paranoia, and mental disorientation are examples of adverse effects that may occur, despite their rarity.

clenching of the teeth, an odd aftertaste, lightheadedness, and a chilling or itching sensation

When a person's eyesight is affected by modestly low blood pressure, symptoms such as headaches and squinting may be present (larger than normal) pupils

irregular or quickening of the heartbeat

Difficulty Keeping Your Sexual Interests Private experiences of ejaculating heat, abnormality, agitation, or drunkenness a state characterized by gloominess, severe frailty, or sadness

Constipation is a side effect that is infrequent, but it is nevertheless possible.

fatigue leading to drowsiness and sleepiness

antibody reactivity in response to antigen

It is essential that you keep track of your development regardless of whether or not you have any little adverse effects so that you can determine whether or not they vanish when your body adjusts to the medication. If they become intolerable, you should seek medical attention as soon as possible. Should major adverse effects develop while using Priligy, the medication should be stopped immediately, and professional medical assistance should be sought out.

How long do the negative effects of Priligy last, if they do so at all?

The negative effects of Priligy might differ from person to person; nonetheless, the majority of users indicate that the symptoms that are most often experienced improve rapidly. It's possible that after some time taking Priligy, you won't experience any of the mild negative effects associated with its use. In the case that they don't, and you're still experiencing symptoms that are troublesome after taking the drug for a few weeks, it's necessary to make an appointment with a medical professional. You should see your physician in the event that any adverse effects persist for longer than twenty-four hours.

The most effective method for counteracting the negative effects of Priligy

Lightheadedness and low blood pressure are two of the Priligy side effects that may occur, notwithstanding their rarity. Before your doctor will write you a prescription for Priligy, they will likely want to check your blood pressure when you are lying down, sitting up, and standing up. They will also want to know whether you have ever had fainting or dizziness in the past. You should not take Priligy if you are dehydrated, which may happen if you have been perspiring significantly, if it has been more than four hours since you have ingested anything, or if you are unwell with diarrhea or vomiting. This will help lessen the chance that you will pass out (being sick)

Be careful to wash down each dose of your medicine with a full glass of water.

Don't go behind the wheel of a vehicle or handle heavy machinery if you're feeling lightheaded, and try not to get up too quickly if you've been lying down or sitting for a long time.

Sit down with your knees drawn up to your chest or lie down so that your head is lower than the rest of your body if you start to feel lightheaded or dizzy. This may prevent you from hurting yourself in the event that you pass out. If taking Priligy causes you to feel lightheaded or dizzy, you should discuss this with your primary care physician.

If you continue to experience any side effects, including a headache, it is recommended that you consume a lot of water and take some paracetamol. It is not recommended to use ibuprofen while taking Priligy unless otherwise directed by a qualified medical professional. If you are experiencing nausea, it is best to take Priligy with food whenever feasible.

If you notice any more unwelcome effects, you should schedule a consultation with your healthcare practitioner as soon as possible.

The very best of the best

Warnings and precautions about Priligy

However, Priligy is not appropriate for everyone. The efficacy of Priligy might be diminished or even rendered null and void by the use of certain medications or conditions. It is not recommended that men use Priligy if they are either younger than 18 or older than 64 years old. Under no circumstances are ladies permitted to take the medication Priligy. You should not use Priligy if you have a history of severe depression or mania; moderate or severe liver difficulties; an allergy to dapoxetine; or if you have ever had an allergic reaction to dapoxetine.

THE END

Printed in Great Britain
by Amazon

20909599R00025